Award-winning writ[...]
of numerous best sell[...]
press as 'the guru [...]
original voice in hea[...]
commitment, she is [...]
reporting. Leslie was born in California, and is the daughter
of jazz musician Stan Kenton. After leaving Stanford
University she journeyed to Europe in her early twenties,
settling first in Paris, then in Britain where she has since
remained. She has raised four children on her own by
working as a television broadcaster, novelist, writer and
teacher on health and for fourteen years she was an editor
at *Harpers & Queen*.

Leslie's writing on mainstream health is internationally
known and has appeared in *Vogue*, *The Sunday Times*,
Cosmopolitan and the *Daily Mail*. She is author of many
other health books including: *The New Raw Energy*, *Raw
Energy Recipes* and *Endless Energy* – co-authored with her
daughter Susannah – *The New Biogenic Diet*, *The New Joy of
Beauty*, *The New Ageless Ageing*, *Cellulite Revolution*, *10 Day
Clean-Up Plan*, *Nature's Child*, *Lean Revolution*, *10 Day
De-Stress Plan*, *Passage to Power* and most recently, *Raw
Energy Food Combining Diet* and *Juice High*. She turned to
fiction with *Ludwig* – her first novel. Former consultant
to a medical corporation in the USA and to the Open
University's Centre of Continuing Education, Leslie's
writing has won several awards including the PPA
'Technical Writer of the Year'. Her work was honoured by
her being asked to deliver the McCarrison Lecture at the
Royal Society of Medicine. In recent years she has become
increasingly concerned not only with the process of
enhancing individual health but also with re-establishing
bonds with the earth as part of helping to heal the planet.

Author's Note

The material in this book is intended for information purposes only. None of the suggestions or information is meant in any way to be prescriptive. Any attempt to treat a medical condition should always come under the directions of a competent physician – and neither the publisher nor I can accept responsibility for injuries or illness arising out of a failure by a reader to take medical advice. I am only a reporter. I also have a profound interest in helping myself and others to maximise our potential for positive health which includes being able to live at a high level of energy, intelligence and creativity. For all three are expressions of harmony within a living organic system.

Boost Energy

LESLIE KENTON

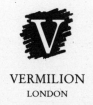

VERMILION
LONDON

1 3 5 7 9 10 8 6 4 2

First published in the United Kingdom in 1996
by Vermilion
an imprint of Ebury Press
Random House
20 Vauxhall Bridge Road
London SW1V 2SA

Random House Australia (Pty) Limited
20 Alfred Street, Milsons Point, Sydney,
New South Wales 2061, Australia

Random House New Zealand Limited
18 Poland Road, Glenfield,
Auckland 10, New Zealand

Random House South Africa (Pty) Limited
PO BOX 337, Bergvlei, South Africa

Random House Canada
1265 Aerowood Drive, Mississauga
Ontario L4W 1B9, Canada

Random House UK Limited Reg. No. 954009

A CIP catalogue record for this book is available from the
British Library

ISBN: 0 09 181440 5

Printed and bound in Great Britain by
Cox & Wyman Ltd., Reading, Berkshire

Contents

Introduction

Lack of energy is the most common complaint of otherwise healthy people. 'I never seem to have enough energy,' they say, 'but what can be done about it?' The answer might surprise you: we all have a great deal more potential energy than we ever use. The key to a high-energy life style is simply a question of learning to tap it.

Maintaining a high energy level is all about balance. It is natural and good to be up some of the time and to wind down at other times. The trouble is that there are some times when it is more convenient to be up or down than others. Too often we treat ourselves like machines and ignore or override the messages our bodies send to our brains.

The *Boost Energy* way is to tune into your body and listen to its needs. Once you understand the way it works and how it is affected by certain stressors, such as food or environment, then you can learn to choose your up times and down times. By maintaining a good balance between the two you'll never reach the stage of complete exhaustion that leads to serious illness.

chapter 1

Feeding the Core

Meet the Energy-drainers

Our world is full of energy-drainers. Excessive noise in cities, environmental poisons in our air and our water, foods and chemicals that we come in contact with – all these drain energy. Their presence in your life, particularly if you have a sensitive disposition, can undermine your vitality – lowering your immunity and making you susceptible not only to colds and flu but also to premature ageing and the development of degenerative conditions.

Energy-blockers, on an external, physical, level can be factors in your lifestyle such as not getting enough exercise, living on a diet of processed foods or eating too much sugar. Over a period of time all three deplete your body of essential minerals and trace elements needed by enzymes to produce energy at a cellular level.

The Energy-drainer Scenario

A woman is in a job which she hates. She feels unmotivated and resentful (*inner energy-drainers*). After work she goes out to drink (*alcohol-addiction drainer*). Sometimes she drinks too much and this creates friction with her husband (*relationship energy-drainer*). She feels bad about herself as a result of arguing (*emotional energy-drainer*). Her poor self-image leads her not to care for herself (*poor self-esteem energy-drainer*). She eats badly (*biochemical energy-drainer*). She feels worse and suffers depression. Nothing in her life seems to work and she has nothing to look forward to . . .

You see the pattern. She is stuck in a rut. The energy-drainers have stolen her personal power and she can only see everything in the worst light.

Now let's look at the flip side. Energy-enhancers tend to attract other energy-enhancers, creating *positive* feedback loops and making you feel empowered and in control of your life. Compare the following situation with the previous sketch.

The Energy-enhancer Scenario

A woman is in a job which she hates. She discovers an inspiring exercise class (*physical energy-booster*). The class makes her feel good about herself and inspires her to eat better (*biochemical booster*). She loses a few pounds, feels better in her body and begins to dress in a more flattering way (*self-esteem booster*). She meets some new friends whose company she really enjoys (*relationship booster*). As her self-esteem increases, the people she works with begin to appreciate her more. Her job becomes more enjoyable (*work booster*). She feels excited about her life and confident about looking for a new job, something she will really love.

Identifying your own blockers and drainers, and

making the choice to let go of even one or two, sows the seed for more positive feedback loops in your life. It is an important step to take in accessing more core energy and developing your personal power. Sometimes even *awareness* itself is enough to get the ball rolling.

Wasting Anxiety

On an internal level few emotions drain energy like anxiety. While you dash about (either physically or in your consciousness) feeling unsafe and unstable and trying like mad to make everything all right, you deplete your body and your creativity. Where there is anxiety there is a high level of electrical, electro-positive magnetic activity and chemical acidity which affect the sympathetic nervous system and encourage feelings of fear, irritability, nausea and headache, as well as an inability to concentrate, muscle pain and insomnia. Even minor attacks of nervousness can dramatically undermine your work performance and make it almost impossible for you to enjoy yourself.

Anxiety is frequently related to food allergies. Re-aligning your diet can help. So can physical exercise which calms electrical and chemical overactivity, replacing it with a more balanced energy, which you can call on, and a feeling of mental and physical wellbeing.

Depression can be a big energy-drainer as well. Sometimes depression develops as a result of blocked emotions which you may not even be aware you are feeling – like grief. Often depression is rather like an anger turned in on yourself to block you from doing harm to anyone else. To break through and release the energy that has been blocked by depression you may need to examine your experience of depression carefully as well as change your lifestyle.

Resentment, too, can be an enormous energy-blocker. Anger immediately felt and expressed keeps energy flowing. As adults we tend to swallow our anger, turning it into resentment. Fear can also block energy. In a measurable physical way it freezes you into inactivity and makes all things seem impossible.

So can negative feedback loops. When you feel low in energy you tend to attract energy-drainers which in turn attract other energy-drainers and before you know it you find yourself caught up in a negative feedback loop. You feel helpless – a victim of circumstances over which you have no power – and you lack the energy or the incentive to break out of the loop.

Core Energy

Being able to call on endless energy depends on how well you feed your core – physically, emotionally and spiritually – day by day. This means developing a lifestyle which incorporates exercise, good food, restorative sleep and the myriad of other possibilities that help support your own brand of vitality at peak efficiency. When creating such a lifestyle for yourself there is one simple but essential thing to remember: your body *is* energy. What your body most certainly is *not* is some dense physical object you have to bolster up or beat into submission so it can keep going.

To create the best possible environment for supporting core energy, fill your life, your home and, as much as possible, your work environment with everything that is life-giving. Sound, colour, light and charged ions in the atmosphere can soothe and restore a system that has been physically and emotionally jangled by a harsh environment. So what resources are available for feeding core energy?

External Enhancers

As the world gets more polluted, the prospect of creating the life-nurturing 'cocoon' of our home environment becomes increasingly appealing. There are many ways to do this. You can draw upon the power of nature to revitalize you, in the form of hydrotherapy and aromatherapy practices, or charge your environment with ionizers, full-spectrum lights, therapeutic magnets and energy-balancing sounds, fragrances, fabrics and colours.

Cool colour

The therapeutic use of colour dates as far back as the first century AD when the famous Roman physician Celsus prescribed medicines of specific colours to treat different ailments. Recent research has confirmed the physiological effects of colour on the mind and body.

- **Red** Stimulating – excites and warms the body, increases heart rate, brain activity and respiration.

- **Pink** Soothing – relaxes the muscles, subdues aggression and anxiety, encourages rest.

- **Orange** Stimulating – encourages appetite and reduces fatigue.

- **Yellow** Energizing – stimulates the memory, increases pulse rate and lifts the spirits.

- **Green** Uplifting – relieves depression, soothes and relaxes both mind and body.

- **Blue** Relaxing – lowers blood pressure, heart rate and respiration; soothes and 'cools' the emotions.

Looking at colour this way can help you create the most appropriate and beneficial colour environments in your home. When decorating your living space, consider which colour qualities are best for a particular room.

Make green friends

House plants can make your home or office environment more friendly and even more healthy. Apart from their uplifting appearance, green plants are also natural air purifiers. Thanks to photosynthesis, they supply a room with fresh oxygen during the daylight hours. Even more important, they can remove toxic organic pollutants from the air. One 12-inch potted plant can clean the air of a 10-foot-square room.

Sleep with a sea breeze

Breathing the air on a mountainside or near the sea makes you feel uplifted and well – 'Ah, good fresh air!' we say. What we are reacting to is the abundance of negatively charged air molecules in each breath. In the city, air pollutants, concrete structures, synthetic fabrics and plastic interiors all conspire to deplete these negatively charged molecules. As a result we can suffer from fatigue, depression and hypertension as well as migraine headaches, allergies and respiratory disorders. A wonderful manmade antidote to polluted air comes in the form of an ionizer – a device which negatively charges air particles. Using one at your office or beside your bed at night can soothe away stress and help you to breathe easy.

Enjoy an air bath

Giving your skin a chance to breathe, unrestricted by clothing, can enhance the body's metabolism and balance body energies. The simplest way to enjoy an air bath is to strip down while you do your morning or evening toilette. Open a window in the bathroom so that there is fresh air. Turn on a heater if the room is too chilly, although cool air for a few minutes can have a stimulating and strengthening effect on the system.

The safe sun bath

The sun's rays, much maligned for their role in the premature ageing of the skin and skin cancer, are also responsible for all life energy on our planet. Without sunlight we would not exist.

The best way to get your daily dose of sunlight is to sunbathe outdoors for carefully controlled periods of time – exposing as much naked skin as possible. Even if the day seems grey and overcast, you can still benefit from the sun's influence. In the summer you should sunbathe only before 11a.m. or after 3p.m. when the sun is not at its strongest. Start with as little as 2 minutes on each part of your body – front, back, left side and right side in full summer sun, then gradually lengthen your time by a minute on each area working up to 10 or 15 minutes on each part per day. This kind of gentle sun exposure, unlike grilling your skin for hours at a time on a sunny beach, will allow you to capitalize on the benefits and avoid the harm of excessive exposure. The use of a total sunscreen on your face whenever you are exposed to sunlight is strongly recommended.

Boxed sunlight

If you spend a good deal of time working in an artificially lit indoor environment you may be deprived of adequate sunlight. Anyone who suffers the symptoms of sunlight deficiency, which can include severe depression, fatigue, and increased appetite and weight gain, can benefit from bringing the sunlight indoors by installing full-spectrum lighting where they live and work or by using a full-spectrum 'light box' every day. Artificial full-spectrum lights stimulate about 90% of the components of natural sunlight, including the UV frequencies. Just a few hours of exposure to them each day has been shown to relieve symptoms of light deficiency in 80% of the cases tested, within only 5 days.

Heaven scent

Not only does scent affect you emotionally but also physiologically thanks to the 'messages' which specific odour molecules carry to your brain. Some of the most powerful message carriers come in the form of aromatic plant oil – the distilled essences of various plants' leaves, fruits, flowers, bark and roots, which are literally brimming over with the structural information of life.

Each aromatic essence carries a different message to the body: vanilla and lavender, for instance, tell the body to relax, while peppermint and rosemary encourage it to wake up. Get to know some of the oils in the list below, and use them to create emotional balance in your environment.

Basil Banishes fear and indecision and clarifies the mind.

Cedarwood cleanses the mind and heightens creativity.

Camomile calms panic and hysteria; good for insomnia.

Clary Sage Clears the head after mental activity.

Geranium Relieves anxiety and depression.

Jasmine Helps counter shyness.

Lavender Calms irritability and impatience.

Lily Restores energy.

Neroli An anti-shock aid, heightens mental functions.

Peppermint Uplifts the spirits; counters apathy.

Rosemary A good nerve tonic.

Sandalwood Helps open the mind to new ways of thinking.

Ylang Ylang An anti-depressant and aphrodisiac.

- Use an essential-oil burner or diffuser to fill your room with energy-enhancing scent molecules. A simple diffuser comes in the form of a ring which you place around a light bulb. The heat of the bulb causes the oils to evaporate into the atmosphere. (But, like any heat-diffuser, it does destroy some of the power of the essence.)

- You can make your own diffuser by putting 8–10 drops of essential oils on a small piece of card-

board or in a dish of warm water and leaving it on
a warm radiator or Aga stove.

● Carry aromatics with you by scenting a handker-
chief with a few drops of oil. You can inhale the
beneficial properties whenever you feel the need,
for instance when you are in a stuffy or smoky
room.

● Keep a collection of a few basic oils such as rosemary, lavender, sandalwood, geranium and neroli
in your bathroom and let them remind you to take
long, soothing aromatic baths. Remember to add
the oils just before you get in (so that they don't
evaporate too quickly). For a normal-size bath use
10–15 drops.

Water wonders
An essential-oil bath can provide you with another
bonus – the restorative properties of the water
itself.

A simple way to incorporate hydrotherapy into
your daily routine is to finish a warm bath or shower
with a 30–45-second cold shower. Doing this first
thing in the morning can set your system into action
for the day ahead or revive you after a relaxing
evening bath and get you ready for a night out.
For extra help, alternate between the warm and cold
2 or 3 times – a minute or two of warm to 30 seconds
of cold – finishing with the cold. It's important that
you wrap up well afterwards, particularly if you are
sensitive to the cold. Daily hydrotherapy can help
improve circulation and make you more resistant to
cold temperatures, but you need to go gently at the
beginning.

Soothing sounds

The final external element is sound. Just as aromatic essences can alter your emotional state, so too can sound. The sound of running water, for instance, winding its way over stones in a stream, has a remarkable ability to cleanse the mind of worries, leaving you feeling calm and clear. The sound of a heart beat played in an infant's cot can reassure her and send her into blissful sleep. You can take advantage of the sounds of nature in the form of cassettes which reproduce the breaking of waves or the calling of birds.

Internal Enhancers

Dynamic people who drive themselves to achieve superhuman feats and continually endure high stress levels eventually burn out and get sick. They ignore one of the most important principles in creating endless energy – the gentle energy of restoration. This can be 10–30 minutes of meditation, a 30-minute afternoon nap or even guided imagery using a relaxation tape. There are also certain days when, for whatever reason, the body just doesn't feel like being pushed. This may be due to the phase of the moon, or the weather or our own biological cycles. It is important to be sensitive to such rhythms and treat yourself with gentleness accordingly if you possibly can. When you do, you discover that these 'soft days' can be full of richness and creativity which goes unnoticed if you are charging around being 'efficient'.

Blissful sleep

The body has its own built-in restoring mechanism – sleep. People who boast about how few hours' sleep they can get away with forget that many essential processes take place during sleep.

Insomnia socks
Next time counting sheep fails, try this instead. Take a pair of short cotton socks and soak them in cold water. Wring them out well and put them on your feet. Then cover your feet with a second pair of dry socks – either wool or cotton – and retire for the night. The cool socks on your feet will help to draw the energy in your body downwards, leaving you feeling calm and relaxed.

Herbal help
Several herbs act as safe and natural tranquillizers which can help relax your mind and body for sleep. One of the most popular is passion-flower or *Passiflora* which can be bought in tablet form. Others include hops, valerian root and skullcap. You can swallow them in pill/capsule form or make a herbal tea nightcap. The classic one is camomile.

Bedtime snacks
Although it is best not to go to bed on a full stomach, some people find it helpful to have a little something before retiring. Some foods help promote sleep whereas other foods taken at bedtime can disrupt sleep.

Good sleep foods
Bananas, figs, dates, yogurt, tuna, wholegrain crackers, nut butter, turkey.

Bad sleep foods
Caffeine, alcohol, sugar, cheese, chocolate, sauerkraut, bacon, ham, sausage, aubergine, potatoes, spinach and tomatoes.

Zen breath meditation

Regular meditation helps improve concentration and focus so that you are able to pour all of yourself into whatever activity you undertake. It can also bring you a better sense of your own centre, providing you with a safe place to return to whenever you feel out of balance. Anyone who experiences erratic energy ups and downs and mood swings can benefit considerably from meditating for 15–30 minutes a day.

Zen breath meditation is one of the simplest yet most effective forms of meditation. Try to meditate for 10–15 minutes to begin with. Keep a watch or clock close by to check on the time.

Sit comfortably and close your eyes. Become aware of your breathing but don't alter it. Watch the breath come in and then out and count 'one' silently to yourself. The next time you breathe out count 'two' and so on up to ten. Then begin again at one. Don't try to change your breathing pattern or anticipate the next number to come. Simply watch the ebb and flow of your breath.

Although it is simple, this meditation, as you will discover, is not easy. It is quite normal for your mind to wander off or for you to lose count. When this happens do not get upset or frustrated. Simply notice that it has happened, smile to yourself and gently bring your focus back to your breathing, beginning again at 'one'. How far you manage to count before you get distracted is unimportant. The numbers are simply a way to help focus your entire being on the breath.

chapter 2

Eating for Energy

Being healthy means a lot more than just not being sick. It means experiencing a sense of grace in your life. It means feeling at *ease*. You sometimes encounter this grace in well-fed young children – children who have been raised on breast milk then given simple wholesome fruits and vegetables, grains and homemade protein foods right from the table. Such a child does not have to stop and consider what she is eating. Provided her taste buds have not been distorted by junk-food and processed drinks, she will quite naturally be guided by her own sense of pleasure and preference and will choose the foods she fancies and therefore the foods her body needs.

Why Eat?

Take a look at *why* you eat. Are you one of a small minority of people who eat just to stay alive but have no real interest either in the taste or the health effects of foods? Is your prime interest in diet from an eating-to-stay-thin point of view? Or do you find yourself worrying most of the time about what and how much you eat so you don't get fat? Or perhaps, you are one of a growing number of people who eat to avoid disease – continually readjusting your eating habits to fall in line with the latest medical report?

Of course all of us are to some extent influenced by most of those food-motivations at one time or another. But to achieve high energy all of the above reasons for choosing foods need to become subservient to one simple goal: eating for performance. In short, you eat because it makes you feel and look great.

Ten Steps to Beat the Energy-breakers

1. Willpower
The first two barriers to overcome concern attitudes, for instance: 'I've tried to give up junk-foods before – but I just don't have the willpower' and 'I know they're bad for me, but I really do like the taste of the "no-no's".'

If you happen to feel this way your 'willpower' is not innately 'weak'. It may surprise you to know that when the old 'should I?/shouldn't I?' conflict arises over a chocolate bar or ice-cream it is quite possible that your reason for wanting it is some sort of biochemical upset in your body such as a deficiency in one or other vitamin or mineral, or just a disturbed digestive system. When your body is in real harmony with itself you are usually indifferent to even the most voluptuous chocolate sundae. So forget the battle of the will. Stop blaming yourself and look to strengthening your overall state of health and raising your energy levels instead.

2. The rewards

One of the most important aspects of any change in lifestyle is being aware of the rewards it will bring you and enjoying them as they arrive. What are the junk-free diet bonuses?

Sparkling eyes and clear glowing skin.

Strong shiny hair.

A firm, well-toned body.

A vanishing pot belly.

A clear mind.

A fresh positive outlook on life.

3. Are you a Mars bar?

One of the greatest incentives to rid yourself of junk-foods once and for all is the startling realization that you really are what you eat as the food you eat becomes the building blocks of the cells in your body. Take a step back next time you are presented with a plateful of chips, sausages and beans and ask yourself, 'Am I really proud to be a greasy chip?'

4. The dreadful cravings

You can't pretend they just don't exist. As Snoopy says, 'It's hard to keep your mind on a diet when your stomach just sent out for a pizza,' so what can you do? Again, take a step back, and acknowledge your cravings for what they really are – you will not die, nor will you even suffer, without that quick junk-food snack, and the sooner you realize it, the better. Then you can take steps to banish them.

5. Substitutes

It's all very well denying yourself this or that, but what do you eat to fill the gap?

Replace refined grain products with wholemeal ones such as bread, pasta, crackers, noodles and rice.

Replace ice-cream and milk shakes with fresh fruit sorbets, frappés and yogurt.

Substitute healthy snacks made by grinding nuts and dried fruit and forming them into little balls for chocolate bars.

With a little imagination and experimentation you will find that giving up junk-food is no sacrifice at all.

6. Exercise

One of the ways to lose your dependency on junk-food and to do away with cravings is to get plenty of exercise. Exercise will quickly rid your body of metabolic waste products, the presence of which make you crave the junk-food.

7. Drink like a fish

Another very helpful way quickly to eliminate toxins from your system is to flush them out by drinking lots of liquids. Spring water is great – it cleanses the digestive tract, liver and kidneys. Unless you practically *live* on a diet of all raw foods, drink at least six glasses a day. Fresh raw vegetable juices are even better for cleaning your cells. Herb teas are very useful too. Apart from having their own specific therapeutic properties they are helpful in taking the edge off your appetite when you crave a certain food or feel like a snack.

8. Snacks

Probably the time when you are most likely to confront the Junk-food Demon is when you decide to 'grab a quick bit to eat' to sustain you between meals, or to replace one. If all you can find for a snack is a chocolate bar or packaged apple pie you are better off going hungry. Missing a snack, or even a meal for that matter, is no terrible sin. On the other hand, if you are hungry, you are hungry. Try to make sure that you have good snacking material at the ready – a piece of fruit or a bag full of crunchy crudités are ideal. Sunflower seeds or unsalted nuts are a good energy sustainer, but make sure they are really fresh and remember they are also high in fat so you may not want to eat them too frequently.

9. Junk the junk

You can't tell every fast-food restaurant to close down or every street vendor to move his cans of fizzy drinks out of your sight, but what you can do is be responsible for the food in your own home. Don't take the attitude that as you bought that large chocolate cake you ought to finish it anyway, and don't let it sit around staring you in the face. Get rid of it, or give it away. The sooner you eliminate 'tempting' foods from your own kitchen, the easier it will be for you to forget about them altogether.

10. Steer clear of the traps

Don't let yourself get into difficult situations socially where you are forced to eat bad foods. Don't be afraid to turn down your Aunt Betsy's trifle – you've probably eaten it enough times to convince her that it tastes OK. Be determined and don't let obstacles such as cynical remarks from onlookers or 'friends' prevent you from reaching your goal.

21st Century Nutrition

When it comes to foods for high-level wellbeing and emotional balance there is one basic principle to remember: *The whole is greater than the sum of its parts.* The best foods are *whole* foods – fresh, natural foods – not foods which have been processed to death. They arrive on your plate and enter your body just as Mother Nature intended them for eating – radiant with their own natural colours and textures.

The real *joy* of eating fresh whole foods lies in their taste, their texture and the remarkable ability they have to bring new life and excitement to a palate which has become jaded.

Cooking starts at the shopping stage. It is when you are in the market surrounded by great mounds of lettuces, avocados, fresh peppers, parsley and squid that you get your inspiration. Never set out to buy food with too fixed an idea of what you intend to buy. Some of the very best dishes can be made from the commonest, least expensive vegetables such as carrots, turnips and watercress and often the cheapest fish is the most tasty when prepared simply. While shopping you may come across something which, although you have not thought of it, is beautiful. It *draws* you to it. Buy it. Forget what you thought you were after. A good menu is created while you shop. Why seek something which is not

Eat for Endless Energy

- Choose the foods you prepare for your meals from the best, freshest you can buy on the market (or better still from those grown in your garden or on your windowsill).

- Choose organic vegetables and fruits when you can find them. Lobby your greengrocer and supermarket to make more available. These foods contain the highest and best complement of minerals.

- Unless you are vegetarian, eat organic meat and chicken. They not only taste better, but have a quite different fat content and come from much healthier animals.

- Eat fresh fruit, preferably organic.

- Eat only whole grain cereals and breads, pasta and crackers, without added sugar or chemicals.

- Eat live yogurt, pure butter and naturally fermented cheeses as well as free-range eggs.

- Use extra virgin cold-pressed olive oil for cooking and salads.

- Eat 2 or 3 tablespoons of cold-pressed flaxseed oil a day or 3–6 tablespoons of raw linseeds mixed into your breakfast yogurt or on your salad. This is all you need to make sure you are getting the essential fatty acids which your body requires for energy and long-lasting health.

- Eat 50–75% of your foods raw – raw fruits and vegetables, organic raw seeds and nuts and grains soaked overnight to break down their hard-to-digest starches. When you are under stress, increase the percentage of raw foods you eat closer to the 75% mark. It is an effective way of creating more energy and balance for yourself when you need it most.

- Grow as many of your own foods as you can yourself. Make 3 or 4 raised beds if you have room in your garden which you close-crop all year round with vegetables. You can grow salad stuff in between rose bushes if you have a small garden. If you have no garden, grow sprouted seeds and grains in your kitchen window or on the sill in the bedroom. They are cheap, easy to produce and lots of fun.

there or out of season? Instead let yourself be tempted by what you find and make it the focus of your menu. Always *seek* temptation. *Food should be so good that it feels sinful.*

Grazing for Energy

The way you eat does not change overnight – nor should it. If you want to create for yourself a high-energy way of eating, do it gradually. Look at the list below and tick any of the steps that are already part of your approach to eating. Then choose a new one to try. See if you can tick off one new step every week. By improving your diet bit by bit you are more likely to see your choices become permanent positive eating habits.

1. Find healthy snack alternatives.
2. Replace ice-cream or puddings with live yogurt, combined with fruit and/or honey for a delicious dessert.
3. Buy yourself 2 or 3 packages of herb tea to try instead of tea or coffee. Some teas are tasty iced. You can fill an empty mineral water bottle with tea to drink chilled throughout the day.
4. If you aren't ready to give up coffee, try organic instead.
5. Wean yourself off sugar and sweeteners in tea or coffee. Instead use honey and decrease the amount gradually.
6. Don't skip breakfast.
7. Replace commercial breakfast cereals with Live Muesli (see p.32).
8. Become an avid label-reader and shun anything containing artificial additives, preservatives, hydro-generated fats and sugars or artificial sweeteners. Check your cupboards, fridge or freezer for any of these items and make a mental note to find an alternative to them the next time you shop.
9. Before you tuck into a leg of deep-fried chicken or a cheeseburger make the mental connection that your body is made of what you put into it.
10. Make a commitment not to eat and run. Even if you are having a snack, eat it sitting down. Chew your foods well and allow your body a chance to digest them before you dash into a stressful activity.
11. Don't eat when you're emotionally upset or anxious, depressed or bored.

12. Learn how to grow your own sprouts.
13. Be *conscious* while you are eating and take time to enjoy the taste, texture and variety of your food.
14. Make 1 meal a day a Master Salad (see p.34).
15. Find an organic source of meat, poultry and eggs.
16. Remove excess fat from meat before you cook it. Remove the skin from chicken.
17. Use skimmed milk instead of full-fat milk.
18. Drink filtered or bottled water instead of tap.
19. When you eat out in a restaurant, avoid items that have been cooked in fat. For instance, instead of fried fish in batter have grilled fish with lemon. Ask for sauces and salad dressings on the side so that you can leave them there if they are too rich or full of junk fats.
20. Vary your diet from day to day always looking for original new dishes to keep your taste buds happy.

Energy Recipes

The following recipes are designed to give you a taste of Eating for Energy eating. You do not have to stick slavishly to the instructions – they are only guidelines. If, for instance, a recipe calls for broccoli and you hate it, you can quite easily substitute cauliflower. The idea is to take the recipes and adapt them to *your* taste, making them your own. A note on quantity: most of the following recipes are designed to feed 2–4 people. As the quantities are approximate, amounts can easily be adjusted to suit your own particular needs.

Where measuring is important the following American measures are used:

1 C = one cup or eight fluid ounces (about the size of a large teacup).

1 T = one tablespoon.

1 t = one teaspoon.

Ultimate Breakfasts

Live Muesli and Energy Shakes are made from foods which are easy to digest, are high in essential nutrients like vitamins, minerals and fatty acids, provide quick energy and will also help sustain you throughout the morning. I often just have a piece of fruit for breakfast, such as an apple, a pear or a bunch of grapes. Fresh fruit is the ideal breakfast for anyone who wants to lose some weight.

Live muesli

This recipe is similar to the original muesli developed by the famous Swiss physician, Max Bircher-Benner. Unlike packaged muesli, which usually contains too much sugar, and is rather heavy and hard to digest, the bulk of this muesli is made up of fresh fruit. It will leave you feeling light and lively.

1–2 heaped T (15–30 ml) oat, rye or wheat flakes
a handful of raisins or sultanas
1 apple or firm pear, grated or diced
2 t (10 ml) fresh orange juice
1 small banana, finely chopped
2 T (30 ml) sheep's or goat's milk yoghurt (optional)
1 t (5 ml) honey or blackstrap molasses (optional)
1 T (15 ml) chopped nuts or sunflower seeds
1/2 t (2.5 ml) powdered cinnamon or ginger

Soak the grain flakes overnight in a little water or fruit juice to help break the starch down into sugars, along with the raisins or sultanas. In the morning, combine the soaked grain flakes and raisins with the apple/pear and banana, and add the orange juice to prevent the fruit from browning and to aid digestion. Top with the yoghurt, then drizzle with honey or molasses (if desired). Sprinkle with chopped nuts or sunflower seeds and spices.

You can prepare countless variations of Live Muesli by using different types of fresh fruit, such as strawberries, peaches, pitted cherries or pine-apple, depending on what's available. When your choice of fresh fruit is limited, use soaked dried fruit, such as apricots, dates, more sultanas, figs or pears. For extra goodness, sprinkle the muesli with a tablespoon of wheatgerm. Wheatgerm, like unsulphured blackstrap molasses, is rich in minerals and vitamins (the B-complex vitamins in particular).

Energy shake
This recipe is best made from sheep's or goat's milk yoghurt.

8 fl oz (1 C/225 ml) plain yoghurt
a handful of strawberries or raspberries
1 t (5 ml) honey or blackstrap molasses
1 T (15 ml) coconut (optional)
a squeeze of lemon juice

Combine all the ingredients thoroughly in a blender or food processor and drink. Depending on the type of yoghurt used, you may need to thin the shake with a little fruit juice.

As with Live Muesli, you can vary the Energy Shake by using different kinds of fruit, such as bananas, mango or fresh pineapple. You can also add extra 'goodies': a tablespoon of lecithin (especially good for slimmers), a raw egg yolk (good for hair and nails) or wheatgerm.

Master Salads

The secret of a Master Salad lies in the following 5 elements:

- **Use the best ingredients** Choose the freshest, most flavourful vegetables you can find.

- **Go for imaginative combinations** Combine complementary flavours and textures for interest – use some ingredients raw and some cooked.

- **Get clever chopping** Create variety by the way you chop, shred, dice or grate. (How you cut a vegetable actually makes a difference to how it tastes!)

- **Make irresistibly delicious dressings** A good dressing can make an indifferent salad great. A great dressing makes a great salad heaven!

- **Add tantalizing morsels** These give a salad its character and often provide not only interest but also substance in the form of protein.

The salad repertoire

The best salads are made from a combination of raw and cooked ingredients. Here are some suggestions.

The raw vegetable line-up

Leafy greens such as spinach, the lettuces – cos, Webb's Wonder, Chinese leaves, salad bowl, frisée, radicchio, lollo rosso, oak leaf, lamb's tongue – watercress, mustard and cress, red and white cabbage, carrots, beetroot, radishes, baby turnips, baby parsnips, celeriac, chicory, fennel, red, yellow and green sweet-peppers, cauliflower, broccoli, avocados, spring onions, mangetout, baby peas, tomatoes, cucumber, courgettes, celery, mushrooms.

The cooked vegetables

- **Sautéed** The following vegetables are especially delicious wok-fried or sautéed in a heavy pan with olive oil before being added hot or cold to the salad: mushrooms, onion, shredded white or red cabbage, mangetout, French beans, courgettes, finely grated beetroot, peppers.

- **Steamed** Although they can also be enjoyed raw, broccoli and cauliflower are particularly nice lightly steamed in a salad. Steamed asparagus and French beans are also tasty.

- **Grilled** Aubergines, sweet peppers, courgettes and fennel, sliced lengthwise and grilled with olive oil and garlic like the Italians do, develop a wonderful flavour.

- **Potato plus** Boiled or baked in their jackets and chopped into salads, potatoes give body and a contrasting soft texture.

Keep extra cooked salad goodies refrigerated in an airtight container to help make 'instant' salads.

Broccoli and hazelnuts

Tear a few leaves of salad bowl or Webb's Wonder lettuce into bite-sized pieces. Lightly steam several broccoli florets. Drain them and slice into bite-sized morsels. Toast a handful of hazelnuts in a frying pan until golden. Peel and dice an avocado. Halve several cherry tomatoes. Place all the ingredients in a salad bowl together with a handful of alfalfa or mixed sprouts and a few leaves of fresh basil. Toss with Spicy Vinaigrette (see p.38) dressing and serve. If the cooked ingredients are still warm, so much the better!

Crunchy potato salad

Potatoes make a comforting and filling salad – especially welcome on gloomy winter days. Coarsely grate 1–2 carrots. Chop 2 sticks of celery lengthwise and then across into small pieces. (In general the smaller you chop vegetables the more flavour they have.) Dice half a red pepper. Chop 2 potatoes cooked in their jackets. Mix the ingredients together with a handful of wheat sprouts and some freshly chopped parsley.

Smooth spinach salad

Made with tender young organic spinach this salad is sheer delight. Tear several spinach leaves into bite-sized pieces. Halve a few radishes. Finely dice half a head of fennel. Finely chop a ripe tomato. Slice several tinned hearts of palm crossways. Dice an avocado. Finely grate 1–2 hard-boiled eggs. Combine all the ingredients in a bowl with a few pitted black olives and toss with a garlic-flavoured vinaigrette dressing.

Stuffed lettuce

iceberg lettuce leaves
2 T soft goat's cheese
1 small carrot, grated finely
2 t fresh chopped herbs
a tiny piece of crushed garlic if desired

Mix the ingredients together then roll up inside the crisp lettuce leaves and serve.

Magic morsels

- **Hard-boiled eggs** Finely grated hard-boiled eggs add texture and body. They are especially delicious in spinach or lettuce-based salads.

- **Toasted seeds and nuts** Put sunflower, pumpkin or sesame seeds, almonds, cashews or hazelnuts into a frying pan and brown them until golden, stirring to prevent them from burning. Add them to almost any salad combination for crunchiness.

- **Oven-roasted sprouts** Place 3–4 day wheat, barley or soya-bean sprouts on a baking tray and sprinkle with sea salt or vegetable bouillon powder. Bake for 15 minutes in a moderate oven. They become crunchy and make delicious sweet salad croutons.

- **Tasty morsels from a tin** Keep the following tins handy to liven up a salad that 'lacks something': sweetcorn (without added sugar), hearts of palm, artichoke hearts, olives, capers, tuna fish (packed in brine), anchovies.

Irresistible Dressings

Choose your salad dressing ingredients from the very
best available. The ultimate is cold-pressed olive oil.
If you can get very fresh walnut or hazelnut oil they
are also a real treat for dressings. Cold-pressed flaxseed oil makes an energy-enhancing addition. Here
is one to begin with, but enjoy making up your own.

Spicy vinaigrette

We use this vinaigrette, or one of its variations,
more than any other dressing. Place the following
ingredients in the bottom of a screw-top jar:

2 t of wholegrain mustard
1 t vegetable bouillon powder
the juice of one lemon or 4 T of cider vinegar
1 t of tamari

Then add one or more of the following:

1 T chopped fresh herbs such as basil, marjoram and
    parsley; or
1 t of finely grated ginger root; or
1 clove of garlic (pressed); or
1 t (heaped) of sun-dried tomatoes or olive paste or
    pesto sauce

Season to taste with freshly ground pepper. Add 1C
of cold-pressed olive oil and shake to combine the
ingredients.

Wonder Sprouts

When a seed, pulse or grain begins to germinate it
becomes a wondrous energy factory producing vast
amounts of essential nutrients.

In just a few minutes a day you can cultivate a continual sprout supply so that you never run out of fresh salad ingredients. One of the simplest ways to grow a variety of sprouts is as a mix. I particularly like a combination of alfalfa with lentil and mung. To this add a few fenugreek or radish seeds for extra zest. Another favourite is wheat sprouts which have a delicious chewy texture and nutty flavour. Sprout these on their own because they are ready so quickly – usually in 2–3 days.

DIY sprout mix

In a large glass jar place 6 T of alfalfa seeds and 2 T each of lentils and mung beans. Fill the jar with water and leave to soak for about 12 hours (or overnight). Drain the excess water away by placing a sieve over the neck of the jar, and then rinse and drain twice more. Divide the mixture between two (or more) jars so that there are no more than two inches of sprouts in each. This way your sprouts will have sufficient room to breathe and grow. Rinse and drain the sprouts twice a day.

Alternatively take a seed tray and line it with paper kitchen towels, then spread the sprout mix over the bottom of it. Simply spray the sprouts with water from a plant spray twice a day and stir them around gently for aeration. After 4–6 days, when the alfalfa seeds have developed little green leaves, the mix is ready to harvest. Rinse the sprouts well and drain. Store them in the fridge in an air-tight container or in sealed polythene bags to be used abundantly in salads and other vegetable dishes.

Sprout burgers

1 C of almonds or a mixture of almonds with sun-
    flower seeds
1–2 C wheat sprouts
2 carrots
2–3 spring onions
1 egg
1 clove garlic
2 t vegetable bouillon
dash of Worcestershire sauce
fresh parsley (finely chopped)
olive oil

Grind the almonds (or almonds and sunflower
seeds) in the food processor and place in a bowl.
Blend the wheat sprouts until fairly gooey and add to
the nuts. Finely grate the carrots and chop the spring
onions. Stir the ingredients together and add the
seasonings. Finally stir an egg into the mixture to
help bind it. Form the mix into patties with your
hands and fry in olive oil. Sprinkle with fresh parsley
and serve. Makes about 12–16 vegetarian burgers.

Soups

Hearty vegetable soup

1 large onion
2 leeks
3 sticks of celery
1–2 carrots
1 turnip
1 parsnip
2 medium-sized potatoes
1 C fresh garden peas or lentil sprouts

2 T olive oil
1 litre of boiling water
1 T bouillon powder
1–2 t herbes de Provence

Wash and scrub the vegetables. Peel the onion. Dice the root vegetables and celery into small cubes and finely chop the onion and leek. Sauté the leek and onion in the olive oil in a large cooking pot. Add the celery, carrots, turnip, parsnip and potatoes and put on the lid. Allow the vegetables to sweat for 5 minutes. Add the boiling water, bouillon powder and herbs and simmer for 30–40 minutes. Add the peas (or sprouts) and cook for a further 15 minutes.

Instant soup
This is ideal when you want a quick light supper.

1 t vegetable bouillon powder
1 egg
1 spring onion (finely chopped)
a squeeze of fresh garlic
a sheet of toasted Nori seaweed or a few toasted
    sesame seeds
a drop or two of Tabasco sauce or a little tamari
boiling water

Stir the bouillon powder into a mug of boiling water. Whisk an egg into the broth with a fork (it will 'cook' almost instantly). Add the garlic and the spring onion. Sprinkle crumbled Nori and/or a few toasted sesame seeds on top. Season with Tabasco or tamari. Drink with the help of a spoon.

You can also make delicious chilled soups, such as:

Gazpacho

4–6 peeled tomatoes
3 carrots
2 sticks of celery
a dash of cayenne

Put through a centrifuge juicer, sprinkle with chopped chives and diced green pepper. Serve chilled.

Snacks
Snick snacks
If you're looking for an alternative to chocolate bars or biscuits to snack on, try this delicious recipe. It combines a quick energy source, in simple fruit sugars, together with sustained energy from nuts and seeds to tide you over between meals.

1/2 C almonds
1/2 C sunflower seeds
1/2 C dried dates
1/2 C dried figs
2 T desiccated coconut
1/2 t natural vanilla essence
1 T malt extract or honey carob powder (optional)

Toast the almonds and sunflower seeds in a frying pan and then grind coarsely in a food processor. Add the dried dates and figs and blend until well combined. Put the mixture in a bowl and stir in the coconut, vanilla essence and malt extract (from health-food stores) or honey. Form into little balls with your hands and roll in carob powder. Refrigerate and enjoy between meals with a cup of herb tea.

Other snack suggestions

● Toasted sunflower seeds and pumpkin seeds.

● Homemade popcorn with a little sea salt.

● Carob Pods (sometimes called St John's Bread – the dried pods can be chewed in place of a chocolate bar.

● Apples.

● Crudités such as carrot, celery and red pepper sticks. Also good for a packed lunch together with a delicious dip.

● Oatcakes (sugar-free) or rice cakes (both available from health-food shops). Enjoy them plain with your tea or juice, or spread with a little butter or nut butter.

● Fresh squeezed vegetable juice (keep in a flask with ice cubes to protect from oxidation).

● Hot spicy apple juice – put concentrated apple juice (available from a health-food shop) in a mug and add boiling water and allspice or cinnamon to taste.

Alternative Drinks

Coffee, if you are a steady 'user', is addictive. Its removal can cause powerful withdrawal symptoms. These usually appear as nausea or a headache lasting from a few hours to several days. But the withdrawal symptoms are worth going through to be rid of caffeine once and for all.

Coffee substitutes

The best substitutes usually don't resemble coffee very much in anything but colour, but nevertheless they can be delicious in their own right. They are usually made from chicory and barley or dandelion root, together with spices, and are good sweetened with a little honey and made with hot milk or hot water topped with milk. Good varieties include Dandelion Coffee, Pioneer and Barley Cup. Hot goat's milk with honey and cinnamon, or with a little carob powder and honey, makes a nice replacement for cocoa. Another good hot drink can be made by adding hot water to a pure concentrated fruit juice such as apple or blackcurrant which can be found in health-food shops.

Herb teas

You can make a wonderful refreshing cup of herb tea using single herbs or herbs and spices in combination. Herb combinations can be found in health-food shops – loose or in sachets. Some of the most delicious single teas include:

- **Peppermint**
  great for settling an upset stomach

- **Lemon Verbena or Lemon Grass**
  both good tonics

- **Camomile**
  calms the nerves

- **Golden Rod (*Solidago*)**
  a good diuretic for those who retain water

- **Lime Blossom or Passion-flower**
  good for relaxing you

Herb-tea tips
The trick of making good cups of herb tea is first to find several herbs or herb combinations which you enjoy and then to add one or several of the following:

● a squeeze of lemon juice or a slice of lemon

● a teaspoon or so of lightly scented clear honey such as acacia or clover

● a drop of goat's milk or skimmed milk (especially nice with spicy teas)

● a dash of powdered cinnamon bark stick

Try making a strong pot of your favourite tea and adding a sliced peach to it. Sweeten with honey, then chill for a couple of hours in the fridge and drink iced in tall glasses.

Eating for Energy: Sample Menu

On rising: A cup of hot water to which the juice of half a lemon has been added, to help alkalinize your system and to promote complete elimination.

Breakfast: Half a grapefruit, a mango, some cherries or other fresh fruit.
A bowl of Live Muesli (see p.32) *or* a bowl of wholegrain porridge with a sliced banana, skimmed milk, a dash of cinnamon and a tablespoon of honey.

Lunch: A large mixed salad of raw vegetables dressed with a light dressing made from yogurt or lemon juice or olive oil and cider vinegar and sprinkled with chopped eggs, sunflower seeds, low-fat cheese or minced chopped nuts. Wholegrain toast if desired.

Dinner: A fresh raw salad of tomato, cucumber and watercress, tossed with plenty of sprouts.

4 oz grilled chicken from which the skin has been removed.

A selection of fresh vegetables such as cauliflower, broccoli or courgettes steamed or wok-fried and served with fresh or dried herbs and spices instead of butter and salt, or added raw to your salad.

A piece of wholemeal Greek pitta bread or a portion of long-grain brown rice, or a baked potato.

Fresh strawberries.

For snacks you can eat fresh fruit, wholewheat rolls stuffed with salad, pitta bread, raw sunflower seeds.

chapter 3

Exercising for Energy

Nothing connects you with your own power like regular physical activity. It brings you in touch with your own body so you experience it as a living breathing organism capable of radical transformation rather than as an object separated from your *self* to be measured against media ideals and found wanting. Exercise carried out with a real awareness of being *in* your body helps to heal splits between mind and body more easily than anything else – the right kind of regular exercise can transform your life.

Energy in Motion

Have you ever started an exercise programme with great enthusiasm – bought a new pair of running shoes, or treated yourself to a gym subscription – only to find that several weeks later you give up? If so you're not alone. Most people who take up a new form of exercise give it up again within a few weeks. Why? Everybody knows that exercise is supposed to be *good for you*. For many this knowledge alone provides the incentive to give it a try. So you buy the gear and dive into activity. You feel inspired and virtuous . . . at least for a while. Then resistance raises its ugly head. Your body aches a bit one day, the weather is bad the next, you get out of the wrong side of bed, you notice how much better the other girls in the aerobics class look in their leotards . . . your enthusiasm wanes and you exercise less and less. Eventually, in spite of guilt pangs, you slip back into the 'comfort' of not exercising.

While this scenario is very common, it is also true that some women who begin to exercise stick at it. Why? Are they blessed with greater willpower? Do they not encounter resistance? Or are they just naturally more athletic? In my experience it is none of these. Anyone can develop willpower, everyone has their off days and anyone can become athletic. The real difference is that the consistent exerciser has been lucky enough to cross from the 'I should' camp of exercisers to the 'I want to' one.

Just Do It

In the beginning we are all in the 'I should' camp. We have to kick-start ourselves into action and it's not easy. However, experiencing some of the benefits of exercising, such as having more energy or feeling good about yourself, can spur you on. If you continue long enough (and 'long enough' is different for everyone), one magical day you find you are actually beginning to *enjoy* yourself. Instead of dreading the next exercise session and fighting the excuses not to do it, you look forward to it. Of course this does not make you immune to resistance or excuses. And you may still stop exercising for a period of time, but because you have experienced the fun of it, something will call you back. Returning to exercise will be easier each time.

If you are afraid to even begin to get in shape, because you feel you are too old, too overweight or just too unfit, remember that the more impossible the challenge of becoming an exerciser seems, the more power for transformation exercise holds for you. Everyone has to begin somewhere.

Why Should I Exercise?

Take a look at the following list of reasons to exercise and circle those you consider to be the 'right' ones.

1. Because it's good for me.
2. Because I enjoy it.
3. Because I'm overweight.
4. Because it lifts my spirits and helps me feel balanced emotionally.
5. Because I look awful in shorts.
6. Because it makes me feel proud of my body.
7. Because most people I know who have their act together do.
8. Because it makes me stronger – better able to cope with stress.
9. Because my friends/lover do.
10. Because it brings me a sense of confidence and self-esteem.

If you circled most of the even numbers then you have begun to understand the concept of living from the core. The odd-numbered reasons are based upon external demands or expectations. They imply an 'I should', i.e. in order to look right in a short skirt or because I have been told that it is healthy or because my friends exercise – I should. The even-numbered reasons, however, all directly relate to core values such as choosing to be whole, to be free and to trust in life. These strong reasons carry core energy and automatic willpower.

Easy Does It

We in the West have this weird notion that if a little of something does you good, twice as much good will come from a double dose. When it comes to physical activity, nothing could be further from the truth. It is low-intensity exercise which is trans-formative, not pushing yourself to your limits or going for the burn. This means exercising at around 70% of your maximum heart rate (MHR) for 30 to 45 minutes between 3 and 6 times a week – not harder (see Your Maximum Heart Rate). It is the same kind of exercise which can be used to exchange body fat for beautifully toned muscles.

Your Maximum Heart Rate

Your target rate for physical activity is 70–85% of your maximum heart rate. Here is how to calculate your own MHR:

Subtract your age from 220. For instance if you are 36 years old, your MHR would be 220 minus 36 or 184. Your ideal aerobic range is then figured by multiplying that number by 0.7 for the low end and 0.85 for the high. For a 36-year-old that works out at 129 to 156 beats per minute. When you are exercising within this range it is considered safe. If you are exercising to help raise your self-esteem, get rid of depression and anxiety or encourage fat loss from your body, you need to exercise so your heart rate stays around the lower figure – 129.

Pulse Test

Here's how to take your pulse during exercise:

After a few minutes of exercising, stop and put 3 fingers over the radial artery at your wrist to find your heart beat. Using a watch with a second hand count the number of heart beats over a period of 15 seconds. Then multiply this by 4 and you will know immediately if you are working out in the right range.

Pick Your Pleasure

Begin by choosing the right activity for you. If you love company then solitary jogging down a country lane may suit you less than joining a gym or taking a dance class with friends. If you are shy and easily discouraged by the idea of exercising in public you might be happiest working out with an exercise video in your home. There are dozens of ways to access core energy through movement. Once you become fit and confident in your body you may be inspired to try the more adventurous or exotic activities – from rock climbing and fencing to flamenco dancing or sky diving. But be careful to differentiate between those which are aerobic and those which, because of their stop-start nature, are not. To be energy-producing, exercise must be steady and sustained. Here is a list of various possibilities (by no means exhaustive) to give you some idea which are aerobic and which anaerobic.

- **Aerobic activities** Brisk walking, jogging, running, rebounding, cycling, dancing, skipping rope, skating, cross-country skiing, rowing.
- **Anaerobic activities** Squash, tennis, golf, downhill skiing, callisthenics, isometrics, weight-lifting.

For the beginner who wants to make exercise a regular habit, walking, rebounding and running are particularly helpful because they are so simple.

Plan Your Schedule

Make an exercise schedule for the coming week. Ideally try to include at least 3, 30-minute sessions of your activity. Begin with 20 minutes and work up to 45 minutes or more. You may like to try a variety of activities such as an exercise class one day, walking another and swimming another. Make time for your exercise by planning in advance. Set your alarm to wake you up an hour early, for instance, or organize a childminder for an extra hour at the end of the day if needs be, so you are free to exercise.

Chart Your Position

Getting fit, like getting anywhere, means knowing where you are setting out from. Use the Pulse Test to work out your present fitness level and establish your ideal workout range. Be sure to exercise at this level for optimal rewards. In a month's time you can retake the test to see your improvement. Another good way to see your progress is by taking a CAT scan. This technique, available at some fitness centres, measures your body fat to lean body mass ratio. It can be really inspiring for anyone who is overweight to see that beneath their fat is a lean muscular body ready to emerge. As you become more fit, burning up excess fatty deposits, chart your success on a follow-up scan.

Paths to Power

One: Walk free

Ideal for anyone who thinks they are too unfit to exercise. Although it may seem like a soft option, in fact walking is one of the very best forms of aerobic exercise. A 6-mile walk burns up only 20% fewer calories than a hard run over the same distance. An excellent choice for anyone who feels low in energy or is convalescing, walking is also particularly convenient because you can incorporate it into your daily routine to get you from A to B.

To begin with decide to walk for 30 minutes a day at a pace where your breathing becomes heavy but not strained. Make sure you wear comfortable clothes and good walking shoes. If you walk to work you can carry another pair of shoes with you to change into. After a week of walking for 30 minutes a day, go a step further. Try walking for an hour and see how far you get. As a guideline you should be able to manage 3 miles in an hour at a leisurely pace. As you become stronger you might like to try hill-walking or even running.

Two: Bounce into shape

Rebounding is the perfect solution for anyone who wants to exercise at home, no matter what their fitness level. Unlike many in-the-home exercise options rebounding has a particularly high continued-use success rate. In case you are unfamiliar with the term, it means bouncing up and down on a mini-trampoline. Apart from being fun, rebounding has some extraordinary health benefits thanks to the forces of gravity exerted on you as you bounce. At the top of each bounce for a split second gravity is non-existent. You experience weightlessness like an astronaut in space. At the bottom of a bounce, gravity is increased by 2–3 times its normal force. This rhythmic pressure on each of your body's cells stimulates the lymphatic system to eliminate stored wastes.

Begin bouncing gently so that your heels barely leave the trampoline. If you feel unsteady, use the back of a chair to support yourself with one arm as you bounce. You might like to bounce to music or even while watching your favourite television programme. As an alternative to bouncing with both feet together, try jogging from one foot to the other. Begin with 10–15 minutes a day and work up to 30 minutes or so as your strength increases. You can also do various exercises on the rebounder to work the muscles throughout your body.

Three: Run to freedom

Ideal for anyone who is keen to experience the high-energy benefits of regular exercise quickly. Running is perhaps the most adaptable and practical of all forms of exercise. For anyone who travels often it can be ideal. Running shoes, shorts and a teeshirt (plus a thin waterproof top and a Walkman if you like) take up minimal space in a suitcase. You can also run almost any time and anywhere.

Since it first became popular, running or jogging has received some bad press with claims that it provoked back problems and other injuries. Minimize injuries by wearing a decent pair of running shoes (not any old plimsolls) and stretching out for 5–10 minutes before and after running.

Begin by making a circuit for yourself of about a mile. Start out slowly and jog as far as you can. Don't push yourself so hard that you are breathless. At the right pace you should still be able to carry on a conversation as you jog. If you do find you get out of breath, alternate running with walking. Above all be patient. After a week or two, see if you can run the whole mile. When this becomes easy, increase your distance until you can run 2 or 3 miles. If you are really ambitious you might like to try a marathon. Experts claim that once you can run for 45 minutes you can begin to train for one.

Power toning

In addition to aerobic exercise, the following exercise routine, based on the Pilates technique, helps to keep the stomach, buttocks and thighs trim. In just 10–15 minutes a day these simple exercises can help sculpt away excess fat, leaving your body strong and toned.

NB: Remember to breathe out during the most strenuous part of the exercise, and in on the recovery. If you are doing a leg lift, for instance, breathe out as you lift the leg against gravity and in as you lower it again. Don't push yourself too hard. Instead work with kindness. Try for 10 repetitions of each in the beginning. As your muscles get stronger, you can increase the repetitions to 20 or more.

Stomach I

Lie on your back with your arms by your sides. Lift your knees into your chest and then stretch your legs up towards the ceiling, toes pointed. Now lift your shoulders and chest off the floor, stretching your hands away from you along the floor. Keeping your chin tucked into your chest, squeeze your buttocks and inner thighs together. Now begin beating the floor with your hands. Breathe in for 4 beats and out for 4 – count 1. Then breathe in again for 4 and out for 4 and count 2 and so forth up to 10. Then rest, hugging your knees to your chest.

More advanced: hold your legs at 60° to the floor instead of 90°, turn your thighs out, flex your feet and squeeze the thighs together.

Stomach II

Lie on your back as in Stomach I. Lift your legs to the ceiling, toes pointed. Lift your chest off the floor, this time reaching your arms at an angle of about 60° to the floor (or think of reaching your hands to the corner where the wall in front of you meets the ceiling.) Holding this position with your upper body, lower one leg towards the floor until it almost touches, then bring it back up. Repeat with the other leg. Do 5–10 with each leg and rest.

More advanced: as with Stomach I, hold your highest leg at 60° instead of 90°.

Waist-refiner stretch

Stand or sit with legs astride. With your hands clasped behind your head stretch over to one side for a count of 10, then to the other side. Repeat 2–3 times on each side.

Waist lifts

Lie on your side with your head resting on your elbow and your other hand in front of your chest on the floor for balance. Keeping your body in a straight line, legs stretched out and toes pointed, lift both feet off the ground as high as possible and lower again. Repeat 10–20 times on each side. NB: Don't be discouraged, this exercise is hard!

Leg lifts I

Lie on your side in a straight line as for Waist Lifts. (If you have trouble balancing, lie with your back against a wall.) Rest yourself on the forearm of your underneath arm, with your hand pointing either in front of you or towards your head. Place your other hand on your upper hip. Bend your underneath leg to a comfortable angle. Stretch your upper leg with the foot flexed and lift it up to about 8 inches above your hip, then lower. Make sure you lift only the leg, not the hip, by using your upper hand to keep your hip still. Repeat 10–20 times on each leg.

Leg lifts II

Lie on your side as for Leg Lift I. This time bend your upper leg and place your foot comfortably in front of your knee or thigh. Place your underneath forearm along the floor as in Leg Lift I, but place your other hand in front of you on the floor for support. Now lift the underneath leg up, toe pointed, and lower. Repeat 10–20 times on each leg.

Leg lifts III

Lie on your side, supported on your forearm as in Leg Lifts I. Place your upper hand on the floor in front of your chest for balance. Bend your underneath knee to a comfortable angle. Now stretch your upper leg, lifting it to the side, about hip level, then swing it forward in front of you to an angle of 90° to your body. Now lift the leg up about 6 inches and lower again to hip level in front of you. Lift and lower in this position 10–20 times and then return the leg to the side and lower. Repeat with your other leg.

Leg lifts IV

Lie on your stomach, supporting your upper body on your forearms, looking ahead of you. With your feet about 8 inches apart, straighten your legs, turn your thighs out and squeeze your buttocks together. Now lift one leg at a time, pulling your stomach muscles up towards your head to support your lower back. Repeat 10 times on each leg.

Thigh lifts

Kneeling up on your hands and knees, stomach lifted, swing one leg out to the side, keeping the knee bent, so that the lifted knee forms a right angle with the one supporting you, and then lower. Repeat 10–20 times with each leg.

For a more difficult variation, after lifting the knee to the side, keep it lifted and move it around to the back as far as possible, then return it to the side position. Move it back and to the side each time. Repeat 10–20 times on each leg.

Cushion squeeze

Lie on your back, with your knees bent, feet together, soles flat on the floor. Place a cushion between your knees. Press your lower back to the floor and squeeze your knees together for a count of 5 seconds. Then relax. Repeat 5–10 times. Finally, with the cushion squeezed between your knees, contract and release your buttock muscles, lifting your pelvis just slightly off the floor as you do. Repeat 10–20 times.

Grab Some Incentive

- Find a picture of your chosen activity or an inspiring quotation (I like 'Just Do It') and pin it up on your bathroom mirror and fridge for encouragement.

- Before you go to bed at night, give yourself a pep talk about your activity the following day and envisage yourself enjoying it.

- Lay your exercise clothes out ready for the next day. Many runners agree that the hardest part of a morning run is putting their shoes on and stepping out of the door. After that it's easy.

- Make a deal with a good friend to get fit together. Sharing the challenge of reclaiming body power with a friend is much more fun.

- If you choose walking or running as your activity, borrow or buy a dog to accompany you. Dogs have endless enthusiasm for walks and runs (however bad the weather).

- Hunt for a good coach or teacher – especially if you choose to work out at a gym or take an exercise class. The right one can provide encouragement and motivation.

You are bound to encounter resistance at some point in the form of injuries, bad weather, illness, or disruption of your routine due to other commitments. Don't chastise yourself and feel guilty about not exercising or breaking your programme. Simply set yourself a date to begin afresh.

Boost Energy

High energy means, more than anything else, an ability to live fully, to give of your very best and to be open to all the good things life has to offer. In many ways it is a little like being a child again, where the colours are so vivid and the world is so full of wonder. Now is the time to take a look at your own energy habits and see if maybe some of them need changing. Then, gradually, you will be able to create for yourself a high-energy lifestyle which in time will become second nature. Once you learn how to tap into the energy within yourself, once you experience how good a high-energy lifestyle can make you feel, energy will never again be something you have to worry about.

Further Reading

If you found this book useful you might like to read other titles by Leslie Kenton. All are available from good bookshops or simply telephone Murlyn Services on 01279 427203. Titles include:

The Dynamic Health Series: a short series of collectibles on every subject – quick to read, practical and life-changing.

● **10 Day Clean-up Plan** (Ebury Press, £6.99)
A step-by-step guide to regenerating your energy while transforming the way you look and feel – all in ten days.

● **Raw Energy Recipes** (Ebury Press, £6.99)
Eating lots of fresh, raw foods can help you look and feel younger, and protect against colds, flu, fatigue and stress.

● **Cellulite Revolution** (Ebury Press, £6.99)
This plan revolutionizes, rebalances and re-establishes a healthy body ecology so you can live cellulite-free forever.

● **10 Day De-Stress Plan** (Ebury Press, £6.99)
Learn how to master stress with a minimum of fuss and a maximum of pleasure. Start now to make stress a friend forever.

● **Lean Revolution** (Ebury Press, £6.99)
Calorie controlled diets don't work. This book shows you how to eat more to shed fat the energy way.

● **Raw Energy Food Combining Diet** (Ebury Press, £6.99)
Food combining is a smart way to shed unwanted fat without counting a calorie and it will make you feel more alive.

● **Juice High** (Ebury Press, £6.99)
Discover how raw fruit and vegetable juices can energise your life, rejuvenate your body, expand your mind & free your spirit.

The Classic Series: each book a bible combining up-to-date scientific research with the time-tested principles of natural health and beauty.

● **The New Joy of Beauty** (Vermilion, £9.99)
Real beauty is nothing less than the full expression of the individual nature of a woman. *The* bible to health and beauty.

● **The New Ageless Ageing** (Vermilion, £8.99)
A marriage of high-tech science and natural health, this book offers a complete anti-ageing programme.

● **The New Ultrahealth** (Vermilion, £8.99)
The latest research into high-energy health allows you to explore the heights of well-being, physically and emotionally.

● **The New Biogenic Diet** (Vermilion, £8.99)
Health, nutrition and permanent weight loss based on natural fresh foods which have been carefully combined.

● **The New Raw Energy** (Vermilion, £8.99)
This meticulously researched work shows how fresh, uncooked foods can work wonders for your body and your life.

Also by Leslie Kenton:

Passage to Power (Vermilion, £9.99)
Few women in our culture are prepared for menopause, nor for the next phase of their life. Exploring the biochemistry and physiology of menopause, alongside myth and archetype, this book will transform the lives of women over 35.

Nature's Child (Ebury Press, £6.99)
How to raise a happy, healthy, independent child the natural way.

Endless Energy (Vermilion, £9.99)
Using simple yet potent energy-enhancing techniques for your body, mind and spirit, learn how to realise your full potential and reach new heights of good looks, creativity and joy.

Index